Real Fertility Diet

How to use preconception nutrition and fertility awareness to get your body ready for pregnancy

Koso Brown

Contents

Introduction

An embryo starts forming its organs and the tissue that will eventually become its brain and spinal cord within three weeks of conception. Most women still don't know they are pregnant three weeks after conception. Therefore, ensuring that your body is in optimal condition is crucial if you intend to become a parent shortly. You are two to three weeks along when you miss your period, which is often the first indication that a woman is pregnant. A baby's heart starts pumping fluid four weeks after conception, and the neural tube—which creates the brain and spinal cord—has already closed.

Your body makes do with what it has to start creating a whole new being. Exercise, body composition, and nutrition are all crucial in getting your body ready for the rigorous demands of pregnancy. The fact that your lifestyle can truly change the genes of your unborn child is even more startling. Put another way, even though their genes are normal, a few specific circumstances make their genes either overwork or not function at all! Balance is key to healthy conception; you need to figure out how much nutrition is ideal for your body. You and your children's health might suffer from both overeating and undernourishment. We will go into great length in this book on the significance of preconception diet as well as other things that have an early impact on the health of both you and your unborn child.

Chapter 1

Preconception health: What is it?

Your health before conception is known as preconception health. Your chances of becoming pregnant can be increased by maintaining good health before conception. When you do become pregnant, it can also aid in avoiding pregnancy-related problems. Receiving a preconception checkup and discussing any health issues that may impact your pregnancy with your healthcare practitioner are important aspects of good preconception health. It also involves making lifestyle changes that could have an impact on the health of your unborn child when you become pregnant, such as taking folic acid to help prevent birth abnormalities.

Start putting your health first at least three months before you start trying to get pregnant if you're considering becoming pregnant. It could take you longer to prepare your body for childbirth if you have medical issues that could interfere with your pregnancy.

What is a preconception checkup?
A preconception checkup is a prenatal medical examination. It assists in ensuring that you are well and that your body is prepared for pregnancy for your healthcare professional. Your doctor can treat and occasionally prevent health issues that could interfere with your pregnancy with the help of this checkup. For instance, before pregnancy, your doctor provides you with any necessary vaccinations and confirms that your immunizations are current. If at all possible, schedule your preconception examination with the medical professional you wish to handle your treatment if you become pregnant. A preconception examination is available at any time. Despite having previously given birth, get one. It's possible that since your last pregnancy, your health has changed.

Why is knowing your family's medical history vital before getting pregnant? Any medical diseases and treatments you, your spouse, and every family member have undergone are documented in your family health history. Before becoming pregnant, it's a good idea to compile your family history so you can discuss it with your doctor when you have a checkup.

The medical history of your family may assist your provider:

- ❖ **Treat health conditions before pregnancy.** Certain long-term, chronic health issues might cause issues getting pregnant and occasionally even birth abnormalities. Treatment for diabetes, hypertension, lupus, and PKU before conception can increase the likelihood of a successful pregnancy and healthy offspring.

- ❖ **Determine any medical issues that run in your partner's or your family's ethnicity.** A collection of individuals who share a language or culture and are frequently from the same nation is known as an ethnic group. Certain genetic disorders, such as Tay-Sachs disease and sickle cell disease, are more prevalent in members of particular ethnic groups. For instance, Tay-Sachs and other genetic disorders are more common in Ashkenazi Jews than in other populations.

- ❖ **Identify the reason for a condition you experienced during a previous pregnancy.** To help determine the source of the problem, your provider may do procedures such as blood tests or ultrasounds. Receiving therapy can reduce the likelihood that you will experience the same pregnancy-related issue in the future.

What is the vitamin folic acid?
Every cell in your body requires folic acid, a B vitamin, for normal growth and development. It can help shield your unborn child from brain and spinal birth problems (also known as neural tube defects, or NTDs) if taken before and during the early stages of pregnancy. Health issues that exist from birth are known as birth defects. Birth defects cause one or more body parts to alter in form or function. They may result in issues with general health, the body's development, or its functionality.

Before you get pregnant, begin taking a daily vitamin supplement containing 400 mcg of folic acid to help prevent NTDs in your unborn child. A supplement is a product you take to compensate for the lack of specific nutrients in your diet. For the first month and a half of your pregnancy, begin taking 400 micrograms of folic acid each day. You can take a folic acid supplement as:

> ➤ A supplement with only folic acid in it.

➢ A vitamin supplement with multiple vitamins. This tablet keeps your body healthy with its abundance of vitamins and other nutrients.

➢ A prenatal vitamin. This multivitamin contains all the elements you require for a healthy pregnancy. Prenatal vitamins are available over-the-counter without a prescription, or your healthcare professional may write one for you.

Even if you're not attempting to get pregnant, you should take a vitamin supplement containing 400 mcg of folic acid daily because nearly half of pregnancies in the US are unexpected.

Take 4,000 mg of folic acid daily if you are at high risk of having a child with neural tube defects (NTDs). Three months before becoming pregnant, as well as during the first twelve weeks of the pregnancy, begin taking 4,000 mcg daily. Find out how to safely obtain this amount of folic acid from your doctor. Taking multiple multivitamins or prenatal vitamins can lead to an excess of certain nutrients that could be detrimental to your health.

You can work with your provider to determine the most effective and secure method of obtaining the recommended daily allowance of folic acid. You run a danger if:

✓ You or your partner has an NTD.

✓ A child of your partner has an NTD.

✓ You previously became pregnant with an NTD.

Additionally, food items such as breakfast cereal, pasta, fortified bread, and tortilla and tortilla chip products manufactured with corn masa flour are good sources of folic acid. To find out how much folic acid is in each serving, read the product label. Several fruits and vegetables are also excellent providers of folic acid. Food that naturally contains folic acid is referred to as folate. Broccoli, orange juice, beans, and leafy green vegetables are foods that are high in folate.

Risks of inadequate diet and health for your unborn child:

✓ Changes in Epigenetics

✓ Miscarriage

✓ Defects in the neural tube (brain and spine)

✓ Heart Imperfections

✓ Lip and palate clefts

✓ Low birth weight at delivery

✓ Fetal alcohol spectrum disorders

The risks of inadequate diet and health:

✓ Depression in pregnancy

✓ Diabetes during pregnancy

✓ Pre-eclampsia

✓ High blood pressure

Chapter 2

Persons' Lifestyle

You and your spouse intend to get pregnant, so it's critical to take the best possible care of your health to ensure that your unborn child has everything it needs to flourish and start growing from the moment you become pregnant. Cell division and formation start as soon as fertilization. After fertilization, your embryo starts to grow its organs in under three weeks. Differentiation is the process by which cells get instructions dictating the kind of tissue they should become before proliferating.

The majority of birth abnormalities happen during your baby's most critical and sensitive developmental stage, which coincides with its time of differentiation and growth. Your kid could suffer irreversible harm if they don't get the right nutrients or are exposed to other dangerous stimuli. It is crucial to get ready for pregnancy in advance because of this. Treat your body as though you are pregnant from the start because many organs and tissues have already started or finished developing by the time you learn you are pregnant. Within ten weeks of conception, the organs of your unborn child are nearly fully formed.

Three weeks after fertilization:

- ✓ Major systems and structures begin developing
- ✓ The brain and spine begin to develop
- ✓ The gastrointestinal tract begins forming
- ✓ Rapid growth occurs
- ✓ Arms and legs begin to bud

Four weeks following fertilization:

- ✓ The structure that creates the brain and spine, the neural tube, is finished.
- ✓ My heart beats and pumps.
- ✓ Facet characteristics start to emerge

Epigenetic and DNA

Spine and bones start to develop The foundation of all living things, including humans, is DNA. In DNA, a blueprint is found. It has all the data and guidelines required to create a singular human being. Every cell has DNA, which it uses to carry out several functions. For instance, the DNA within a pancreatic cell instructs it on how to produce the hormone insulin. Upon fertilization, the sperm and egg combine to form a newborn, whose DNA is quickly formed and present in each of the baby's millions of cells. It was long believed that DNA could never be changed.

It is now understood that although the information in DNA cannot be altered directly, it can be altered. **The term "epigenetics" describes how environmental factors alter DNA function.** Your body serves as the environment for your unborn child since it is where they develop. Bacteria, chemicals, food, and stress are a few elements of the environment you give your child. Consequently, some sections of your DNA may be "turned on" or "turned off" as a result of all these factors. Think about DNA as written instructions.

Certain lines of instruction can be hidden with a whiteout, and other lines can be highlighted to draw attention to them. The instructions are simply covered or highlighted rather than being altered in any way. This is how DNA gets "turned on" or "turned off." Your body's environment employs vitamins, minerals, sugar, fat, stress, and a host of other substances to alter your unborn child's DNA similarly.

This is how, particularly in those initial weeks of pregnancy, the foods you eat have a significant impact on the health of your future child. Pregnancy brings about several permanent and reversible alterations. Pregnancy-specific vitamin and mineral requirements must be met by maintaining a balanced diet, which is crucial for your baby's overall health and well-being as it develops and approaches adulthood. Preconception and perinatal nutrition will hopefully gain momentum as a result of our growing knowledge of the health of unborn children and their impact on the mother and baby before, during, and soon after pregnancy.

Chapter 3

Nutrition

Depending on the stage of pregnancy, diet both before and during pregnancy is extremely complex and ever-changing. Nutrition during pregnancy is hard but crucial since vitamins and minerals are little molecules that naturally interact with one another in the body. It's not difficult to picture the millions of minutes and complex processes that take place inside of you and demand more nourishment when you consider the human being that is developing inside of you. All the nutrients you eat provide the building blocks for the development of your baby. You may provide the ideal groundwork for an ideally healthy baby by eating a well-balanced diet and taking supplements as needed! It is genuinely yours to hold.

There are two primary components to nutrition:

1. Macronutrients
2. Micronutrients

Macronutrients

The three dietary components that you require in significant proportions are referred to as macronutrients. Protein, fat, and carbs are the three macronutrients. It's critical to maintain a healthy balance of these macronutrients throughout your life, particularly if you intend to become pregnant. You are establishing the framework for a healthy pregnancy by ensuring a balanced and healthy distribution of carbohydrates, protein, and fat. Another essential part of a healthy diet is water, which is especially vital during pregnancy when women's blood volumes expand and they require more water to meet this demand.

The carbohydrate

Dairy products, fruits, vegetables, grains, and starches are examples of carbohydrates. They should make up half of your total calories. The quality of the carbohydrates you eat is more significant than obtaining 50% of your calories from them. Select carbohydrates that are high in fiber and natural nutrients and low in fat, salt, and added sugar. Pick a whole-wheat bread with five grams of fiber instead of a white loaf with less than one gram. Fiber not only helps to maintain appropriate cholesterol levels but also slows down the rate at which sugar enters your bloodstream. When selecting a fruit or vegetable, prefer vibrant, dense varieties over light, fluffy ones, such as a carrot over a potato.

Limiting your intake of added sugars is crucial because it has been demonstrated that they adversely and epigenetically alter your developing child.

Fats

Make up thirty percent of your daily calories from fats. Fat comes in three different forms: trans, saturated, and unsaturated. 20% of calories should come from unsaturated fat, and the remaining 10% should come from saturated fat. Trans fats must be avoided at all times.

Unsaturated fats:

- ✓ Avocado
- ✓ Seed and nut oils
- ✓ Additional vegetable oils
- ✓ Canola oil
- ✓ Olive oil

Saturated fats:

- ✓ Additional animal fat
- ✓ Butter
- ✓ Lard
- ✓ Coconut oil

Omega-3s

Another kind of fat is omega-3 fat. Flax seeds, chia seeds, walnuts, fatty fish, and fortified foods all contain it. The growth of your baby's brain and a portion of its eye tissue depends on omega-3 lipids. It also aids in determining gestational duration and preventing perinatal depression. Omega 3 fats should be consumed by pregnant women in amounts of 200 mg per day or 1200 mg per week. You can accomplish this by eating 1-2 servings of salmon, mackerel, or trout each week, or by consuming 1 tablespoon of flax seed or flax seed oil each day.

Complete Protein

Protein is a crucial part of a body's pregnancy preparation and ought to make up at least 20% of daily calories. Eggs, beans/legumes, fish, poultry, meats, and high-protein yogurts like Greek yogurt are examples of foods high in protein. Since protein is needed to develop the placenta and fetal tissues early in pregnancy, it is crucial to consume adequate amounts of it. If a woman exercises regularly or has an extremely active lifestyle, she should eat extra protein. Undernourishment in protein during pregnancy may also result in epigenetic changes that lead to increased fat storage in the progeny throughout their lifetime. This indicates that a low-protein diet during pregnancy increases the risk of obesity and other health issues in the progeny.

Micronutrients

The various dietary ingredients that are still necessary for your body to function but in reduced quantities are referred to as micronutrients. For instance, you probably wouldn't consider slicing up a baguette of pure calcium, but you are aware that sipping a glass of milk will provide your body with part of the necessary calcium. Minerals and vitamins are the two primary types of micronutrients.

Vitamins:

- ✓ Vitamin A

B Vitamins:

- ✓ Thiamin
- ✓ Riboflavin
- ✓ Niacin
- ✓ Pantothenic Acid
- ✓ Vitamin B6
- ✓ Biotin
- ✓ Folic Acid (Folate)

Vitamin B12

- ✓ Vitamin C
- ✓ Vitamin D
- ✓ Vitamin E

✓ Vitamin K

Minerals:

- ✓ The trace element choline
- ✓ magnesium
- ✓ Calcium
- ✓ The trace element iodine
- ✓ Zinc
- ✓ Copper Iron

Everything related to this will be covered in detail below.

Vitamins

Vitamin A:20% increase

Early in pregnancy, vitamin A is crucial because it aids in the development of the heart, eyes, hearing, and limbs of the developing embryo. When cells start to multiply and take on their designated purpose in the third week following conception, it also becomes significant. Because it strengthens the immune system and treats iron deficiency anemia, vitamin A is extremely crucial for mothers.

Even while vitamin A is crucial, taking too much of it in supplement form has been linked to birth abnormalities. Birth abnormalities and naturally occurring vitamin A in food are unrelated. A woman's daily intake of supplemental vitamin A should not exceed 3,000 IU. It's crucial to read food labels for any hidden vitamin A fortification as many foods have extra vitamin A added to them. Because of this, if you choose to take a supplement, make sure the dosage is no more than 1,500 IU of vitamin A. Another unrecognized source of vitamin A is skin care products. Pregnancy should not be planned and skin treatments containing retinoid or retinol should be stopped many months beforehand.

Carrots, sweet potatoes, mangoes, and peaches are among the orange and red foods that are high in vitamin A. Broccoli and spinach are among the dark green vegetables that are abundant in it.

Folic Acid: 147% increase

You can use folate and folic acid interchangeably. Due to its part in the formation of the neural tube, it is one of the most significant vitamins. It is crucial to start taking folic acid supplements if you intend to become pregnant since the neural tube closes four weeks after conception. Your body uses a lot of folic acid 20 days after conception, therefore it's critical to remain replete during this time.

Spina bifida and anencephaly are neural tube abnormalities linked to inadequate folic acid intake. It is also connected to heart problems, limb abnormalities, cleft lip, and cleft palate.

The ideal way to prepare for pregnancy is to take 800 mcg of folic acid daily as a supplement. The body does not absorb natural forms of folate well.

Increase in biotin: uncertain

The fetus uses a lot of biotin, which is broken down more quickly and has declining amounts throughout pregnancy, for a lot of rapid cell division. Early in pregnancy, low levels of biotin can cause teratogenesis, an abnormal development of the fetus that can result in several birth abnormalities. A woman may not be aware of her biotin deficiency because it is not always evident and may not show any symptoms. As a result, taking 30 micrograms of biotin daily as a supplement is safe. It's crucial to always read the label because many multivitamin products do not include biotin.

Liver, egg yolks, chocolate, almonds, and various vegetables are natural sources of biotin. Smaller levels of biotin are found in other forms, but the liver is the main source.

Vitamin B12: 40% increase

B12 is necessary in the early stages of pregnancy. Adequate quantities of this vitamin are crucial because it is one of the most critical factors in the lasting transformation of the baby's epigenetic makeup. Low birth weight babies, neural tube malformations, and other birth problems are linked to Vitamin B12 deficiency. There is an intriguing correlation between folate and vitamin B12. Supplementing with folate can conceal a B12 deficiency and shield a woman from exhibiting any symptoms or indicators of a deficiency. Because most pregnant women take supplements and folate is equally crucial, it is simple to conceal a vitamin B12 shortage.

Since vegetarians and vegans may only naturally obtain vitamin B12 from animal sources, they must take supplements. Other individuals, such as those who have undergone gastric sleeve or bypass surgery, may also experience problems absorbing vitamin B12. Certain experts advise taking a vitamin B12 supplement containing 6–30 mcg or including a daily grain or cereal fortified with the vitamin in one's diet. This would guarantee sufficient absorption for appropriate epigenetic alteration and the avoidance of birth abnormalities.

Vitamin E and C: increases of 25% and 67%, respectively
Both vitamins C and E have strong antioxidant properties. If your diet consists of a variety of colorful fruits and vegetables and is well-balanced and healthful, then you don't need to take supplements. There is simply a slight rise in their needs. But if you smoke, you and your unborn child benefit much from vitamin C and E. Smokers should try to give up the habit and start taking vitamin C and E supplements.

Increase in vitamin D by 300%
The hormone known as vitamin D may be crucial for the growth of your baby's brain, lungs, motor skills, and other organs. The vitamin has a variety of interactions since it functions as a hormone in the natural world. Studies indicate that vitamin D may interact with vitamin A during fetal development, in addition to its known interactions with calcium for absorption. Maternal depression, pre-eclampsia, fewer first-trimester miscarriages, and a host of other conditions have all been linked to vitamin D. It is now widely regarded by specialists as "the miracle vitamin."

Since vitamin D is fat-soluble, your body cannot simply excrete the excess vitamin that is not being used. It is crucial to ensure that you are not overdoing supplements because of this. Before becoming pregnant, it is okay to take a 2000 IU vitamin D pill to help your body become ready. Deficiency is a prevalent condition without any symptoms. It has been demonstrated that approximately 50% of pregnant women are vitamin D deficient.

The best source of vitamin D is cod liver oil; food is a relatively poor supply. Most other foods contain little to no vitamin D unless they are fortified. Your body can truly produce vitamin D on its own when exposed to sunlight because it is a hormone. For women, this varies based on a variety of factors, including skin tone, sunscreen use, location, season, and many more. Therefore, it is advised to take a vitamin D supplement before becoming pregnant if you are not exposed to sunshine for longer than ten to fifteen minutes each day.

Minerals

Calcium: a 122–167% rise

Supplementing before or during pregnancy is not recommended, even though the amount of calcium required increases during pregnancy. Although preeclampsia and hypertension have been demonstrated to decrease in certain trials, calcium supplementation is not necessary during the preconception stage. The growing embryo or fetus does not require additional calcium. Enough calcium should be obtained through a diet high in dairy products or dairy substitutes enriched with calcium.

Iron: 150–180 percent rise

During pregnancy, iron is a particularly vital mineral. It is in charge of delivering oxygen to every part of your body, including the growing fetus, during pregnancy. The fetus cannot grow and develop normally in the absence of sufficient iron. Low iron levels lead to incorrect DNA modification, which makes iron an essential epigenetic modulator.

Worldwide, approximately 50% of pregnant women experience an iron deficiency during their pregnancy. From 15–18 mg to 27 mg per day, needs to rise. Pregnant women nationwide consume only 15 mg of iron on average, which is almost half of the recommended daily intake of the mineral. **"Nearly half of all pregnant women around the world are iron deficient during pregnancy."**
Due to iron's involvement in growth and development, it's necessary to ensure that your levels are appropriate before

conception, even though iron supplementation becomes critical later in pregnancy. With an average of 3 mg of iron per 3-ounce serving, beef is a healthy source of iron. Fish, poultry, and chicken have far lower iron content—roughly 1 mg per 3-ounce serving. At about 5 mg per serving, beans and lentils have a relatively high iron content; however, depending on the kind of bean, this amount may vary. You can easily determine if the foods you eat contain iron because iron content is always listed on the back of food labels.

Consuming enough iron through food alone may be challenging because pregnant women require 27 mg of iron each day. To obtain one day's worth of iron, for instance, you would need two servings of spinach, three servings of beans, and one serving each of beef, chicken, and fortified bread. Consuming enough iron through food alone may be challenging because pregnant women require 27 mg of iron each day. To obtain one day's worth of iron, for instance, you would need two servings of spinach, three servings of beans, and one serving each of beef, chicken, and fortified bread.

For this reason, a 30 mg iron supplement is advised. It will ensure that your present stocks of iron are sufficient for conception in addition to meeting your higher needs throughout pregnancy. It's crucial to remember that iron supplements prevent the body from absorbing zinc. As a result, it's crucial to take zinc supplements in addition to iron supplements.

Zinc: 44% increase

Zinc is necessary for cell division and multiplication in the weeks leading up to conception as well as for the prevention of birth abnormalities early in pregnancy. While non-pregnant women only require 8 mg of zinc daily, pregnant women require 11–12 mg. 82% of women's diets do not contain enough zinc.

Copper: uncertain rise

Zinc should always come first since too much zinc might lead to a copper shortage. Since it is uncommon for a copper shortage to result from a diet deficient in sources, interactions between other vitamins are the primary cause. One classifies copper as a trace element. This indicates that your body requires relatively small amounts of it. But in the absence of copper, several health issues could surface. Copper is employed in the early stages of development in infants and has been linked to the growth of several organs and tissues, including the neural tube. Low birthweight newborns and birth abnormalities are thus linked to copper deficiency.

It's crucial to take a copper supplement or select a prenatal vitamin that contains copper if iron and zinc supplements are being taken.

A 12% rise in magnesium

Magnesium contributes to neural tube closure and early pregnancy development of the embryo. A higher incidence of birth abnormalities has also been linked to magnesium deficiency. These are a few of the explanations for the significance of this mineral in the very early phases of pregnancy.

During pregnancy, a woman's daily magnesium intake should rise by 40 mg to 350–360 mg. Fortunately, many different meals include magnesium. Some of the best foods that contain magnesium are almonds, spinach, soy milk, beans, and cereals. You might be getting adequate magnesium if your diet is well-balanced and includes fruits, vegetables, nuts, and legumes or beans. Nevertheless, 56% of adults still need to consume the recommended amount of the mineral each day. A magnesium supplement is advised if these items aren't a large part of your diet.

45% rise in iodine

Iodine deficiency is thought to be the most prevalent preventable cause of mental retardation worldwide. Iodine is crucial for the early development of the embryo. The synthesis of thyroid hormone and the growth of your baby's brain and spinal cord are significantly influenced by iodine. It also contributes to the development of the anatomical pathways that facilitate rapid brain-to-body communication. Infants who do not get enough iodine are far more likely to experience hypothyroidism, birth abnormalities, and cognitive impairments. Cognitive impairments and hypothyroidism are related. The mother's thyroid hormone production requires iodine. The fetus uses thyroid hormone to create the structures necessary for rapid brain-to-body communication.

Thus, sluggish brain and body function is brought on by low thyroid hormone. The main cause of cretinism, which is why iodine is so important before conception and during pregnancy, is this.

Pregnant women should take in 220 mcg daily, while non-pregnant women should take in 150 mcg. To make sure they get the necessary daily allowance of iodine, women should take a 150-mcg iodine supplement. Salt that has been iodized is the main source of iodine. You might not be getting enough iodine from your diet if you frequently use sea salt or kosher salt. Seaweed, dairy products (if the animals are fed iodized meals), eggs, fortified cereals, and cod and other shellfish are some more major sources of iodine. For instance, you would need to eat one 3-ounce portion of cod, one cup of yogurt, and two eggs to obtain enough iodine in your diet without salt.

If you intend to get pregnant, you should start taking supplements because iodine is crucial for fetal growth even before the mother realizes she is carrying a child. Recognizing that the majority of prenatal supplements are devoid of iodine is crucial. Thus, remember to always read the label on any prenatal vitamins you buy.

Choline: undefined rise

Women should consume 450 mg of choline daily because it is crucial for the early development of the fetus's brain. In the early phases of pregnancy, it is also a crucial nutrient for the development of organs, cell division and multiplication, and cell   differentiation.

Babies born to women with sufficient choline may develop cognitively more advanced cognitive abilities. Studies on animals revealed that rats with high choline levels in their moms had higher memory and spatial awareness. Numerous foods, such as pork, eggs, and wheat germ, contain choline. The liver should be avoided during pregnancy due to its unusually high vitamin and mineral content.

Chapter 4

Foods to Limit or Avoid in a Fertility Diet

Everybody will have a distinct fertility diet, therefore when it comes to nutrition, it's crucial to constantly listen to your body. However, it could be useful to know how the following meals can affect your fertility if your goal is to become pregnant. In this manner, you may make empowered food decisions.

Caffeine

If you enjoy your morning cup of coffee, you don't have to give it up totally, but it might be beneficial to drink tea and coffee in moderation when attempting to conceive. While drinking tea or coffee doesn't appear to interfere with ovulation15, it may promote dehydration.

According to gynecologic surgeon Angela Chaudhari, MD, an assistant professor in the Department of Obstetrics and Gynecology at Northwestern University Feinberg School of Medicine in Chicago, "Our morning cup of coffee is the worst thing we can do from the standpoint of dehydration." Caffeine is also a diuretic, which means that it can keep your mucous membranes from remaining wet, which could change the consistency of your cervical mucus. (The sperm have a better chance of "sticking" to and reaching the egg if you have more viable cervical mucus.)

It could be a good idea to start this practice now as the American College of Obstetricians and Gynecologists (ACOG) advises pregnant women to keep their daily caffeine intake—from coffee, energy drinks, teas, and even chocolate—to under 200 mg.

Rather, think about cutting back on your daily caffeine intake with herbal teas, decaf coffee, and other low- or no-caffeine beverages. For example, a Nutrient study discovered that green tea may enhance fertility. Green tea has less caffeine than an equivalent cup of coffee or brewed black tea, even if it isn't entirely caffeine-free (an 8-ounce cup of brewed green tea typically has between 30 and 50 mg). Herbal drinks like hibiscus, ginger, and chamomile teas are further low- or no-caffeine possibilities.

Processed Soy

Because soy may have a detrimental influence on fertility, it may be advisable to avoid forms of processed soy in your fertility diet, especially powders and energy bars. For example, a study published in the Journal of Nutrition discovered that diets heavy in soy can have a deleterious effect on ovarian function. Some experts think that these products' high levels of soy protein isolate have estrogen-mimicking qualities that can throw off your hormone balance.

Take note that fermented soy products like miso paste or natto, as well as whole soy products like edamame and tempeh, are OK in moderation. "When we're eating soy in its most natural form like in other cultures like Japan and China, it's great for the body.

Sweetened beverages and artificial sweeteners
Living a balanced life that includes occasional pleasures is crucial. However, sticking to less-processed sweeteners may be helpful if you have any problems with unstable blood sugar levels (for example, if you have diabetes or PCOS) to help increase fertility. Concentrated amounts of sugar can completely upset your blood sugar balance, which can lead to problems with insulin and your whole hormonal balance.

For your fertility diet plan, eat pastries and candies in moderation, but also keep in mind sugar bombs that are more covert, such as fruit juice, energy drinks, and sweet teas. A study published in the journal Epidemiology found that sugared beverages in particular have been linked to ovulatory infertility.

Reducing your sugar intake does not include substituting artificial sweeteners with other products. Select less-processed sweeteners with lower glycemic loading, including agave syrup, honey, maple syrup, or stevia, a naturally occurring zero-calorie sweetener, if you want sugary foods.

Liquor

The majority of experts advise against alcohol consumption for couples trying to conceive. Not only can it cause dehydration, but excessive alcohol consumption—including binge drinking—has also been linked to lower fertility. There may also be certain risks to the fetus if you habitually drink and become pregnant without realizing it.

It's also critical to remember that not only does not drinking help the person who is becoming pregnant; a study that was published in the International Journal of Environmental Research and Public Health found that alcohol use can harm sperm and may have long-term consequences for the developing fetus. In summary? For the time being, it could be advisable for you and your spouse to limit alcohol if you're trying to get pregnant.

Chapter 5

Additional Healthful Recipes

The composition of the body

Your body's makeup affects your baby's development as well. Overweight women may experience issues with the absorption and storage of vitamins and minerals. An infant's likelihood of becoming obese as an adult might also be epigenetically modified by an overweight or obese body. Underweight women are more prone to underfeed their growing pregnancy or give birth to underweight babies.

Every woman should try her hardest to get a normal body weight before getting pregnant. Using an online calculator, you may find your BMI, which should fall within the normal or healthy range. Although your weight-to-height ratio is taken into account by BMI, other factors such as high muscle mass may cause your BMI to be higher than normal.

Work Out

Your body is under a lot of physical stress throughout pregnancy. It's crucial to engage in regular physical activity, especially strength training and weightlifting, to prepare for pregnancy. Reducing the burden that carrying a small human around puts on your body can be achieved by strengthening your muscles and stretching them to increase mobility.

Health Screening and Genetic Testing

Pregnancy preparation also includes getting screened for diseases and performing genetic tests. Your doctor can suggest a genetic panel if there is a family history of a genetic abnormality. It might be especially advised for women of Jewish descent to get genetic testing.

Before getting pregnant, it's crucial to get further health exams for rubella (German measles), thyroid hormone levels, blood type, and CBC for anemia. Make a screening request if you are at risk for any sexually transmitted infections, such as syphilis, hepatitis B, or HIV. It's critical to have a blood test to check for certain STIs before becoming pregnant because they can be passed from mother to kid and may create issues throughout development.

Chapter 6

Tips for an Effective Fertility Diet

When attempting to conceive, it can be beneficial to incorporate other nutrition suggestions into your daily routine in addition to the specific meals you're eating. A healthy body is essential for a good pregnancy and healthy baby, and healthy food lays the foundation for this!

Learn which diets are optimal for male fertility.

It's simple to overlook the fact that a man contributes 50% of the total to the childbearing process. "I'm not saying treat your partner like a child, but if you cook and eat at home together, help make veggies a focus on his plate,". suggests that to stop testosterone from being converted to estrogen, male partners should eat foods high in zinc, such as sunflower seeds and asparagus.

Perhaps to improve male fertility, they should also pass on the cheese plate: Poor sperm motility and concentration have been related to high dairy consumption. Additionally, you can motivate children to take vitamins every day. The prenatal vitamins available in the market are packaged with vitamins that are beneficial to male fertility, such as zinc, selenium, lycopene, C, and E.

Also, Brazil nuts are the best source of selenium, which is excellent for sperm motility. Hold a large bowl that your partner can easily open. Oysters are an additional superfood. In addition to its purported aphrodisiac qualities, the bivalves are high in zinc, protein, and vitamin B12.

Take your vitamins

Consume a daily multivitamin with 40–80 milligrams of iron and at least 400 micrograms of folic acid. Folic acid lowers the incidence of some birth malformations of the brain and spine and encourages the development of the neural tube in babies, according to the Centers for Disease Control and Prevention (CDC). Starting prenatal vitamins as soon as you start attempting to conceive is advised by some specialists.

Select whole foods instead of processed ones. If you want to put the power of healthy foods to work in your life, you could find inspiration in the Mediterranean lifestyle. Whole grains and vegetables are staples of the Mediterranean diet, along with less processed meat, which may help prevent ovulatory dysfunction. Studies have indicated a connection between fertility health and the Mediterranean diet.

Know when you are fertile

While following a fertility diet can aid in conception, scheduling your pregnancies appropriately is also crucial. Because you can only become pregnant during a limited period each month—the day of ovulation and the five days prior—many couples keep track of their reproductive window. Use the ovulation calculator below to determine the optimal time for you to become pregnant.

Conclusion

All women who intend to become pregnant are advised to take supplements of folic acid, which is one of the most vital vitamins. It's also crucial to consider how iron, zinc, and copper interact. Iron supplementation is crucial since pregnant women have significantly higher requirements for the mineral; however, doing so also increases the need for zinc and copper. Because excess vitamin A supplementation has been linked to birth abnormalities, be wary of it in meals and skincare items.

Naturally occurring vitamins, from food do not carry the same risk and should be an essential part of any woman's diet planning for pregnancy. Although nutrition is already difficult, it quickly becomes even more difficult when it comes to getting ready for pregnancy. The dilemma escalates immediately when you learn that the food you eat can alter your baby's DNA because these alterations are frequently irreversible. Nevertheless, eating healthfully before getting pregnant can be a challenging yet rewarding experience. Making the most of your health is the first move. A healthy mother is the foundation of a healthy child, after all.